PUNs and DENs ©

Discovering learning needs in general practice

PUNs and DENs©

Discovering learning needs in general practice

Richard Eve
General Practitioner, Somerset

Foreword by

Professor Janet Grant
Director
Open University Centre for Education
in Medicine

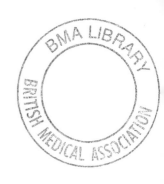

Radcliffe Medical Press

Radcliffe Medical Press Ltd
18 Marcham Road
Abingdon
Oxon OX14 1AA
United Kingdom

www.radcliffe-oxford.com
The Radcliffe Medical Press electronic catalogue and online ordering facility.
Direct sales to anywhere in the world.

British Library Cataloguing in Publication Data

A catalogue record for this book is available from the British Library.

ISBN 1 85775 807 2

Typeset by Acorn Bookwork, Salisbury, Wiltshire
Printed and bound by TJ International Ltd, Padstow, Cornwall

Contents

Foreword

Richard Eve stands out among the array of doctors writing about medical education for his ability to remain first and foremost a clinician. Not for him the rhetorical pastures of educational jargon and theory which so belabour clear thinking about exactly how doctors can best continue to learn. Not for him a primary focus on external managerial or procedural demands, though he enables doctors to comply with them.

Richard Eve has simply looked at what doctors actually do to derive useful and relevant learning based on their daily practice and he has turned this into an elegant system that has been tried and tested. Identifying the Patient's Unmet Needs (PUNs) and the consequent Doctor's Educational Needs (DENs) describes professional development at its most important and useful.

It is a happy fact that PUNs and DENs are ideally suited to the processes of appraisal, personal development plans and revalidation that doctors must participate in from now on. It is an equally happy fact that PUNs and DENs match up to any modern educational imperatives. Managers and educational theorists will have their honour satisfied. But PUNs and DENs were not designed for those purposes. Richard Eve makes it clear from the outset that he has developed this system to suit himself as a doctor who, like other doctors, wants to improve his practice efficiently, effectively and enjoyably, and for no other reason.

This book will enable any doctor to derive pleasure and professional satisfaction from a manageable approach to continued learning – and if you feel that you do not have the time, Richard Eve, the ultimate professional pragmatist and problem-solver, will suggest solutions to that as well. This book is written by a man who not only understands learning but understands how medicine works as well. It is a singular achievement to meld the two.

Professor Janet Grant
Director
Open University Centre for Education in Medicine
February 2003

About this book

With yearly appraisals and General Medical Council revalidation upon us, every general practitioner needs a good personal development plan (PDP). This book outlines one way to create just that. It starts in the consulting room by looking for the Patient's Unmet Needs (PUNs), and then goes on to define the Doctor's Educational Needs (DENs). Richard Eve takes you through the whole process from empowering yourself to take charge of your own learning to putting together a PDP of which you can be proud. This book takes learning out of the lecture theatre and into the realities of day-to-day general practice with a no-nonsense and practical approach.

About the author

Richard Eve is a full-time general practitioner in Somerset and has many years of experience as a GP trainer and clinical tutor. He first piloted his PUNs and DENs system of learning in Somerset in 1994. Since then it has been widely adopted across the UK and abroad, from Australia to Romania, and it is now an established educational tool for discovering learning needs. Richard Eve has run workshops and lectured across the country on self-directed learning. He writes for medical journals and the public alike.

Acknowledgements

Thanks are due to CMP Information Ltd for allowing the reproduction of some material previously published in *Pulse*, and to Dr Roger Crabtree for his excellent cartoons.

Introduction

This book is not written for academics or educationalists. I hope that I have avoided using the jargon that so often makes simple things sound complicated. The book is aimed at the busy general practitioner who is struggling to find time for learning. If just one reader ends up motivated or rescued from 'burnout' it will have been worthwhile. This book reminds you why you need to continue learning (to be a good doctor) and who you do it for (yourself).

Chapter 3 on discovering learning needs with PUNs and DENs, describes how to discover your learning needs from reflection during consultation. If you want to ask your patients directly, then Appendix 1 gives the address to write to for well-tried and tested patient questionnaires. Appendix 2 describes a method that we have used in our practice by asking our peers and colleagues what they think that we might need to learn. It is perfectly safe and unthreatening. If you just want a light and entertaining read, stick to the chapter on reflective practice – an easy read that is designed to drive home the message of how important it is that we find time to reflect on what we do. I make no apology for including a short chapter on exercising caution when assessing 'evidence' and the difficulties that we face in turning our knowledge into something useful. The last chapter outlines how PUNs and DENs can form the foundation for your personal development plan (PDP). The aim of the book is to encourage doctors to take responsibility for their own competence, but there is adequate material in this book to help you to build up evidence to compile a quality PDP that will more than satisfy the requirements of yearly appraisals and revalidation.

Above all, *PUNs and DENs* is designed to put some fun back into learning and to put the GP back in charge of his or her own learning agenda.

Chapter 1

Why bother with learning?

Competence

My reason for learning is so that I can become and remain a good or 'good enough' doctor. I want to be confident, reflective and fulfilled, and enjoy what I do. This is my motivation for learning. I am not driven to learn by demands from outside agencies such as the General Medical Council or primary care trust. So what makes a good doctor? It is not that difficult to define, but it is very difficult to measure. I need to know what skills make a good doctor so that I can focus my own learning and development appropriately. And which skills are the most important ones, that should take most of my time?

Several skills are listed below. Put the four most important ones on the left and the less important ones on the right.

Empathy and sensitivity
Audit skills
Communication skills
Clinical knowledge
Drug budget management
Conceptual thinking
Protocol design skills
Health promotion skills

How did you get on? It is frightening that we seem to be spending what little time that we have for learning on drug budgets, audits, protocols and health promotion. Important as these may be, we must continually upgrade and hone the more important skills first.

Who should we ask to define competence in a doctor? Should we ask our patients, the general public, politicians, the Royal College of General Practitioners, the General Medical Council or perhaps our fellow GPs?

A group of occupational psychologists have made an effective stab at defining what makes a good doctor. They asked a large number of GPs to name a GP who they would be happy to recommend to a friend or to have care for their own family (i.e. they asked someone 'in the know', but from a patient's perspective). They selected those GPs who were most commonly mentioned and put them into three groups. The GPs had to bring with them one example of an incident that they thought represented excellent general practice and one that represented poor general practice – that is, real events that had occurred in general practice. A system was used to identify common themes. The outcome was that 14 different aspects of competency were defined. Thirty-five respected working GPs were facilitated in discovering how to break down and identify the constituents that make a good doctor.

The 14 competencies were as follows:

- empathy and sensitivity
- personal organisation and administrative skills
- communication skills
- personal attributes
- conceptual thinking
- personal development
- managing others

- team involvement
- stress coping mechanisms
- legal, ethical and political awareness
- professional integrity
- job's relationship to society and family
- clinical knowledge
- learning and development.

The language that was used to describe these competencies was encouraging. Phrases included the following: able to compromise ... showing sensitivity to colleagues ... knowing when to delegate ... being aware of own limitations ... having an interest outside medicine ... having humility and empathy ... learning to say sorry and control one's anger ... integrity, flexibility, unselfish, innovative, motivated ... taking responsibility ... able to judge what is important ... respect for those whom society does not like ... keeping up with current practice ... a skilled negotiator ... a good facilitator ... a team player ... willing and able to learn from experience.

This work was later combined with two other methods of assessing competence, namely studying video consultations and asking patients, and the final outcome was published in Patterson F, Ferguson E, Lane P *et al.* (2000) A competency model for general practice: implications for selection, training and development. *Br J Gen Pract.* 50: 188–93.

Clearly, measuring competence is a little more complicated than looking at your beclomethasone/salbutamol prescribing ratio! If you want to ask your colleagues how they judge your competence and see your strengths and weaknesses, I have described a system that we have used in our practice in Appendix 2. If you want to find out what your patients think of your competence, then the address to write to in order to obtain a well-tested and tried system is given in Appendix 1.

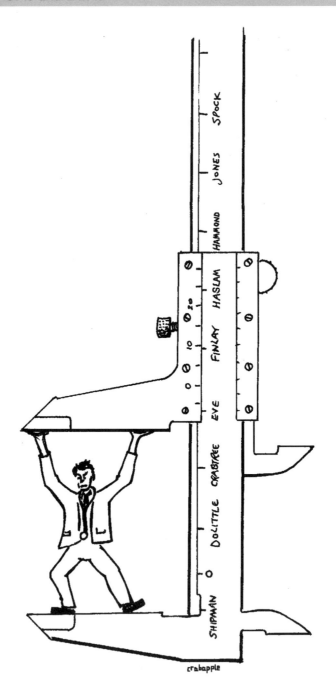

Measuring competence is complicated.

Competent doctors apply evidence-based medicine (EBM). Is the best doctor the one who has got the highest number of heart failure patients on to ACE inhibitors?

Rate the competence of the following doctors.

- *Doctor A.* Identifies and recalls all patients with heart failure. The computer search reveals that he has achieved his standard of 80% of such patients being started on an ACE inhibitor (compliance rates and later treatment withdrawals not recorded).

- *Doctor B.* Is desperate to stay within her prescribing budget. If she goes over budget, the in-house physiotherapy service will be withdrawn and her patients will suffer as a result. She cannot possibly prescribe more ACE inhibitors and remain within budget. She knows the evidence but chooses to ignore it.

- *Doctor C.* Has no direct access to echocardiography facilities. It takes at least six months to see a cardiologist. Personal experience causes him to believe that up to a quarter of heart failure patients will not tolerate effective doses. He feels that if he is to prescribe safely he needs to offer regular follow-up in order to check blood pressure and renal function and to titrate up to the maximum tolerated dose. He feels uncomfortable launching such a programme without the support of secondary care, and since they seem to be overloaded already, and he is busy enough as it is, he elects to postpone the introduction of an ACE-inhibitor-prescribing policy.

- *Doctor D.* Having been made aware of the evidence, she opportunistically reviews her patients when they attend, concentrating only on those who were already on diuretics for presumed heart failure. She takes into consideration compliance, contraindications, the ease with which the patient could attend the surgery and the patient's health philosophy. She is aware of her own over-cautious approach to drugs (and her drug budget), but tries not to let it influence her prescribing. A year after starting her programme a computer search shows that only 30% of her heart failure patients are on ACE inhibitors.

- *Doctor E.* Is very busy organising his colonic cancer screening programme and providing a GP endoscopy service. He has little interest in cardiology and has never heard of the evidence about ACE inhibitors. He continues to practice uninfluenced by this evidence.

What outcome measure will tell you about the competence of these doctors? Prescribing statistics will tell us little. Evidence-based medicine only offers statistical significance relating to cost-effective interventions on 'freak' populations. The good general practitioner assesses its relevance to their own practice population and then translates it into personal significance for individuals in the consultation. In order to do this effectively, a doctor will need attributes in all 14 competencies. Make a start by conducting a self-assessment of the 14 competencies. Politicians are going to need to know that competence cannot be judged on the basis of simple outcome measures alone.

Accountability

Whenever I have come across a patient satisfaction survey, the results have always shown that patients were happy with the service they received and that they had confidence in their GP. Following the Shipman case, the Bristol paediatric cardiology inquiry and the case of a rogue gynaecologist, politicians and the media have expounded the need for the public to be reassured about the competence of doctors. The NHS Executive, Royal College of General Practitioners, General

Practitioners Committee and General Medical Council have had a field day commissioning reports, playing politics, arguing, releasing press reports and setting up committees. So far they have managed to worry the public and make GPs feel threatened and vulnerable. Clinical governance is now well established, and yearly appraisals and revalidation are upon us. Well, don't worry – get your priorities right and all will fall into place.

Place the following in order of priority when it comes to being accountable.

Primary care team
Government
Self
General Medical Council
Primary care trust
Partners
Family and life outside general practice
Patients

I expect that your answers are pretty similar to my own.

Self

Before anything else, you are accountable to yourself. By definition, a professional is someone who is accountable to him- or herself for maintaining competence. Every day doctors make decisions and judgements in the privacy of the consultation. If a doctor loses the inner drive to 'do a good job', then no amount of outside accountability will correct the problem. So it is important to be reflective about your work, think about what you need to stay competent and enthusiastic, and base your learning on your own fulfilment and not on pleasing others.

Family and life outside general practice

Workaholics seldom stay the course. It is vital to programme time for other things, whether they be personal relationships, children, hobbies or other intellectual pursuits. Many young doctors now follow 'portfolio careers'. When you are on your deathbed, do you think your last words will be 'I wish that I had spent more time at the surgery'?

Partners

Dysfunctional partnerships are not uncommon. You are the directors of a small business that is providing care to the same community. How can you do a good job if you are all pulling in different directions? The arguments for a salaried service are gaining strength, but the reality is that most of us are in partnerships and we are accountable to each other. What a recipe! Put together a group of men and women of different ages and backgrounds, with different aspirations and values, and at different stages in their lives, and expect them just to get along fine! In fact, this is a classic example of turning a threat into an opportunity. All of those differences can be turned into a great strength, but not without effort. You will need tolerance and listening skills, you will need to dedicate time to teambuilding, and you will need to discover each other's strengths and learn how the practice can use them. Facilitated 'away-days' can help enormously here.

Primary care team

So you are looking after yourself – you have a reflective, competent, balanced life – and the effort put into achieving a united partnership is paying off. You are nearly there now. We work with a host of other professionals, and primary care is now truly multidisciplinary. We now have an enormous and disparate group that has to work effectively as a team. If the partnership is dysfunctional, what hope is there for the wider team? Nevertheless, we must accept that we are accountable to the whole team, every member of which has aspirations, learning needs and problems that need to be addressed. We used to have primary care team meetings (what a bun-fight!) with 30 or 40 people talking in little groups all at the same time. They didn't last long. A primary care team actually consists of a complex relationship of groups, subgroups, inner groups, loose-knit groups, communication structures and networks. For such an organisation to run efficiently, it needs quality management. I may have a role as a director, but the co-ordination and communication structures are the responsibility of my practice manager. It is a time-consuming job that requires special skills, and by delegating to effective management I am recognising my accountability to the team as a whole.

Patients

Doctors have always been accountable to their patients, if only to protect their reputation. However, accountability is no longer held only on an individual basis, but is now also for the health status of populations. You must address issues not only of empathy, sensitivity, communication skills and clinical knowledge, but also of audit, benchmarking and public health issues. The involvement of patients in the assessment and delivery of care is something that we can expect to see much more of in the future.

The profession

The General Medical Council is no longer limited to removing rogues and the grossly incompetent, and it now wants a bigger slice of the action. The GMC want to play a role in raising standards generally, and believes that revalidation will achieve this.

Primary care trust

You may have grown accustomed to demonstrating some accountability to the health authority with practice reports, referral and prescribing data, but primary care trusts (PCTs) are taking this a step further with clinical governance. Some PCTs may take the enlightened route and view clinical governance as an opportunity to facilitate and support you in your personal endeavours to be a good doctor who is accountable to yourself, your practice and your patients. Other PCTs may take the other route and bombard you with targets, protocols, guidelines, formularies and their chosen audits focusing only on central Government directives. Will PCTs beocme bogged down by controlling budgets and pushing Government National Service Frameworks, or will they be your advocate for the delivery of care at the coalface?

It should not be necessary to regard revalidation and clinical governance as threats. Avoid seeing them as more paperwork and performance measurement and instead view them as no more than a slight irritation. Concentrate on being accountable to yourself, your practice and your patients. You can use PUNs and DENs to create your own personal development plan and professional practice development plan. When the Government, primary care trusts and General Medical Council want some accountability, share just enough of these to keep them happy. Remember that when it comes to accountability, first and foremost you are accountable to yourself.

Chapter 2

Finding time for learning

We want to learn for ourselves, we have our priorities right and we are not going to be intimidated by assessment of simple outcome measures, but how are we possibly going to find the time for any learning?

Suggest anything new to a GP and you can guarantee that the main obstacle to its introduction will be 'I don't have the time or the resources'.

Where is the time to learn?

Integrating your learning into daily practice and discovering your true learning needs is going to take time. Imagine the busy overworked GP, bogged down by clinical and administrative demands, whose patients are clamouring at the door, complaining that they can't get an appointment to see him or her for at least a week, when I roll up and say 'What you want to do is cancel Thursday afternoon surgeries. Shut the surgery and bring back early closing. Thursday afternoons are now dedicated to learning. Welcome to the future of general practice.'

You can imagine the replies: 'Can't possibly find the time',

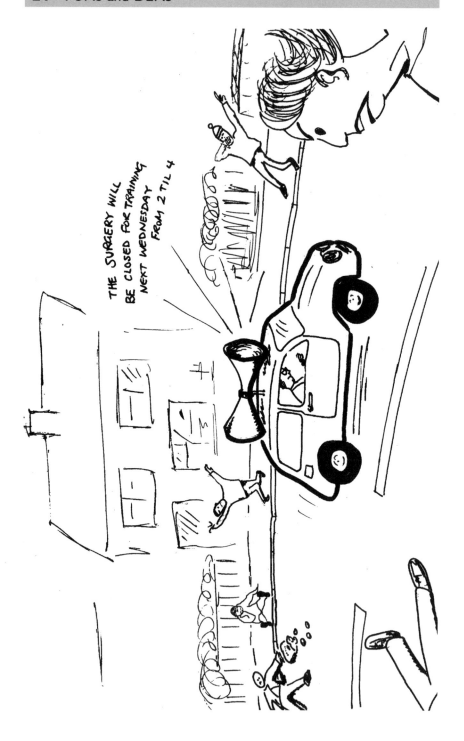

'Far too busy', 'What about my patients? They already find it difficult to get an appointment', 'When will I do my paper-work?', and so on.

Make learning part of the job

In the future, general practice is going to be about quality, not quantity. Just look outside medicine for a moment. In industry, training is not a 'tack-on' of 30 hours each year when one can find the space, but is built into the routine and made part of the job.

Look at hospitals, for example. Since Calman, every department has had to have a full half-day every week for education and training. The continuing medical education (CME) requirements of hospital consultants are double or three times those of GPs, and they only need to know about one speciality. A GP has to know about all specialities as well as their own, and be sufficiently skilled to run a small business.

Keeping up to date

We work in an environment of continual political, organisational and professional change. Clinical knowledge and advances develop at a staggering rate, and patient expectation and demand flourish. It almost defies belief that GPs attempt to stay competent and up to date without dedicating time for reflection, learning and planning.

We are living dangerously. It is time to make a choice either to struggle to maintain availability and expose yourself to the risk of making mistakes because you are too tired, burnt out, non-reflective and ignorant, or to change your priorities and make education more important. You can't be sued for learning, but you can be for poor quality consulting!

Box 2.1: Creating time for learning

Stage 1. Accept that time for learning is a priority.
Once you have accepted that time must be found for learning, and have recognised its importance, you are halfway there. If you don't believe it, then there is no point in going on to Stage 2, which is to devise the strategy for bringing about the change.

Stage 2. Make arrangements for cover while the practice is closed.
The easiest way is just to do it. Put up a notice in the waiting-room, advertise on the repeat scripts, give it a couple of weeks and then close on Thursday afternoons.

That just leaves emergency cover. If you must, take it in turns for a partner to carry a mobile phone, but it is better to reach an agreement with a neighbouring practice to cover each other's learning half-days or, if one is available, to use your local co-op or deputising service.

You have now created breathing space where you can share clinical medicine in the practice. Time is now available to you during the day (instead of last thing at night when you are tired) to build up your portfolio, create your practice development plan, design an audit or receive computer training.

Challenges to overcome

'We can't possibly provide fewer appointments'

Review the consultations, and find out how many were there because the doctor asked them to come. Are you using unnecessary follow-up? Are you using two or three consultations instead of one because you were too tired or ineffective to do it properly in the first place? Are you using practice nurses efficiently? Do you have a telephone consultation system? Do you advertise NHS Direct? *Do you need a notice in the waiting-room saying 'No consultations on Thursday afternoons'?*

'Part-time partners find it difficult to attend'

Review your timetable and rota. Diary management is a challenge to be met, not an excuse for inactivity.

'It will cost us money'

I bet it doesn't, but monitor the items of service (IOS) payments and find out whether it does.

'The health authority or primary care trust won't approve the changes in availability'

Give them a business plan explaining how the quality of care will improve.

At one meeting in London, a GP stood up and told me that his patients would die if he was not there for them. I wonder how they coped at weekends. Did he ever have a holiday? Patients are put at risk if their doctor is exhausted, burnt out, stressed and unhappy. Doctors must take control of their timetable, their learning and their availability.

A major change such as this needs to be owned by the whole practice. The best way to introduce the change is have an 'away-day' and explore all of the issues. I strongly recommend that you employ a skilled facilitator, and be assured that you will achieve a result.

Chapter 3

Discovering learning needs with PUNs and DENs

If we can accept that the primary reason for continual learning is to enable us to remain a good doctor and that, above all, we are accountable to ourselves, we are ready to discover what our true learning needs may be.

Adult learning

Medical education has come a long way. It is much more sensible to talk about *learning* rather than teaching. You may receive a lot of teaching but not actually do any learning at all. Adult learning is relevant to the learner and is learner centred. It is problem based and interactive. Adult learning builds on the learner's personal experience, provides feedback and encourages a desire for further learning.

Learning with PUNs and DENs fulfils all of these criteria. It takes very little time and costs no money – an attractive proposition to GPs! The system ensures that your learning is directly linked to improving patient care. It will also improve your consultation skills. You will discover not only your own

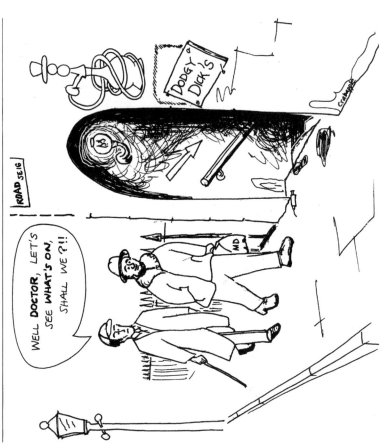

'The master detective was one of the first to make the connection between **PUNs** and **DENs**.'

education and training needs, but also changes that you may want to make within your practice as a whole. Learning with PUNs and DENs is incredibly simple – perhaps too simple for the academics. If you share it with colleagues it can also be great fun.

Box 3.1: Wants and needs

Patient's wants

Patient's needs

Consultation...................Transaction

Doctor's needs

Doctor's wants

I confess to not being very interested in what the patient wants. If it is my job simply to give patients what they want, it does seem a waste of all my years' training and experience if I am there simply to respond to demand. A patient may want a wonder pill to cure their headaches, but you may discover that what they really need is to come to terms with a failing marriage. I am very happy to bring the patient on board. I want us to work together and I want to understand my patient, but the ultimate judgement about their real needs requires as much input from the doctor as from the patient.

Nor am I interested in what the doctor wants to learn. It is natural to take the easy path. We instinctively attend meetings on subjects that we like and already know much about. In the days of PGEA courses, one year I completed my full year's quota entirely on cardiology, which I enjoy. However, my time would have been better spent learning gynaecology, which I don't.

So we can't discover what we need to learn by asking the patient or the doctor what they want. However, we can discover what the doctor needs to learn by exploring what the patient's real needs may be. This process occurs during the consultation (or any other patient interaction). By focusing on the patient's needs we shall discover consultations where we recognise that we have failed to meet the patient's needs. We shall than have found a *patient's unmet need* or *PUN*. At a later date we can then ask ourselves what it is that we need to learn in order to ensure that next time we will be properly equipped to meet that need. We shall then have defined a *doctor's educational need* or *DEN*.

PUN = Patient's Unmet Need
DEN = Doctor's Educational Need

How to do it

The system is not designed as a simple logbook for collecting PUNs whenever something crops up. You can add to your logbook in this way, but it means that you are only collecting PUNs that come easily to mind – ones that you like! The exercise is best carried out as a practice with all doctors and nurses participating. You should select a full week for collecting PUNs. During that week, after every consultation you must ask yourself the following question: 'Was I equipped to meet the patient's needs?'.

In order to answer this question, you will need to have concentrated during the consultation on what the patient's needs might be and whether they were met. You will soon find your first PUN. Of course, more often than not you will be meeting the patient's needs. Inexperienced doctors (e.g. registrars) will collect plenty of PUNs, and more experienced doctors will find fewer of them. Older doctors who are getting weary may find very few indeed because they have lost the ability to be reflective about their work.

Once you have found a PUN, you must decide whether you are dealing with an area of clinical knowledge, non-clinical knowledge, skill or attitude. You are now in a position to define a doctor's educational need or DEN. General practitioners cannot possibly be omnicompetent, and many PUNs will not be met by fulfilling DENs, but by delegation to someone else.

The process can be summarised as follows.

- Spot the PUN
- Define the DEN
- Meet the PUN by either:
  - delegation
  - DEN fulfilment
  - practice management.

DENs can be met by individual learning, but it is better if they are shared either with others in the practice (*in-practice learning*) or to bring agenda to *self-directed learning groups*.

Examples of spotting PUNs and identifying DENs

1 *Clinical knowledge.* A patient with a history of peptic ulcer is seen, who has heard of triple therapy and requests it. You blind him with science, prescribe, and the patient leaves satisfied and impressed. However, only you know that what he actually received was your best guess. Which

is the best combination of antibiotics? Should you have tested for *Helicobacter pylori*? Should he have been referred for gastroscopy? You recognise that the patient's need would have been better met if your clinical knowledge was better (PUN identified and DEN defined). Enter this in the log – that you need to learn more about triple therapy.

2 *Non-clinical knowledge.* The patient's needs may not be met fully because you are unable to tell them when the genito-urinary clinic is open, who is the best surgeon for referral of patients with impotence, who is the duty chemist tonight, etc., as well as where the practice nurse has hidden the speculum, or because you can't find any fluorescein.

3 *Skill.* A patient presents with persistent tennis elbow that needs injecting. You are unable to do this (PUN easily identified and skill DEN defined).

4 *Attitude.* A young man presents with *'can't cope'*, anxiety and tearfulness. It transpires that he has been badly treated at work and is afraid that his job may be at risk. You recognise that you felt very irritated during the consultation, and that instead of focusing on his needs you concentrated on your own need 'How can I end this consultation and move on to the next one'? You may recognise that you have a personal difficulty in dealing with 'wet' men and that your true feelings were 'stop being so wet, pull your socks up, men don't cry, I wouldn't behave like that'. You have identified an attitude DEN that needs to be addressed.

5 *Practice organisation.* A consultation may not have been as successful as it might have been either because the patient was ill prepared (e.g. 'I have been waiting for over an hour and have another appointment to go to' or 'you are very hard to get – I had to wait a week for this appointment') or because the doctor may be ill prepared (e.g. feeling tired

and grumpy because he was up half the night on call (or at a party!), or because he was running behind and unable to keep up with appointment times).

Meeting the PUN or fulfilling the DEN

1 *Clinical knowledge* (triple therapy). A simple need for clinical knowledge. You may go to the library and ask the librarian to help you find an appropriate review article or do a CD-ROM search. You may want to discover local hospital policy and write to your local gastroenterologist and ask him to outline his management protocol.

2 *Non-clinical knowledge.* Some non-clinical gaps in knowledge will be best met by delegation or ensuring that appropriate information resources are available within the practice.

3 *Skill DEN* (elbow injection). You may choose to delegate and meet the PUN that way, or else you could learn the technique. If you choose the latter option, there may be a suitable minor surgery course coming up. You could set up a training session in the practice if others also want to learn the technique, and apply for a PGEA as for in-practice learning.

4 *Attitude DEN* ('wet' men). Recognition and admission of an attitude DEN is educational in itself, and consultations should improve as a result. If the attitude DEN is very restrictive, it may be reasonable to delegate (e.g. if you don't believe in abortion, refer all requests for termination of pregnancy to a partner). There are a lot of 'wet' men about, so it is probably unreasonable for a GP to delegate all such patients, and you should therefore address the issue. You may choose to discuss the problem with colleagues or

partners, but it is better to discuss such issues with a trained educationalist, and a GP tutor may have an important role here. Together you may work out a strategy for recognising and using emotions that are experienced during consultations.

5 *Practice development.* PUNs may follow poor consultations when the problem lies in practice organisation. While building up a log you may frequently identify PUNs because you are too tired or too stressed to give of your best. It will be clearly demonstrated to you that patient care is suffering as a result. The log will need to demonstrate how you respond. You may make changes to your appointment or on-call system and subsequently find that you are identifying fewer Puns due to tiredness or stress.

The logbook: what to record

It is vital that the whole educational process is linked to improved patient care and remains relevant to our daily practice. Each time a PUN is identified, the log should include patient details (name, age and sex). For example, you may find that most PUNs are found in a particular age group. You need to relate your learning need to a particular clinical situation. The discovery side of the log is totally confidential to the individual doctor.

- *Discovery*. Date ... patient identification (name, age and sex) ... describe the PUN ... define area for improvement, development or change ... classify into relevant areas – knowledge clinical (KC), knowledge non-clinical (KN), skill (S) or attitude (A).
- *Process*. Outline the educational plan – define personal

DEN, practice development plan, etc. Record what practice changes, audits or developments you have instigated as a result.

You have now produced a rather smart personal development plan. You have outlined what you plan to do, and it is all linked to improving the care of your patients.

At the back of this book you will find a brief summary of what to do and a logbook for recording your findings. You can photocopy this first for further use after you have filled it up!

Some guidelines and examples

The use of PUNs and DENs in Somerset has been assessed and discoveries have spread across the whole range of problems encountered in general practice. The greatest benefit seemed to be the opportunity to share PUNs within the practice and to share educational needs. Learning with PUNs and DENs stimulated enthusiasm for organising in-practice learning. Practice nurses were equally enthusiastic, and their needs were found to be the same as those of the GPs. The exercise has worked well with doctors and nurses learning together.

Strike rates (the ratio of number of PUNs found to number of consultations) varied enormously, ranging from 2% to 45%. Reasons for low strike rates included the following:

- not bothering to record small PUNs
- a PUN being identified but also being solved there and then in that consultation either by referring to books or by using the telephone. This occurred when the doctor was not

stressed and had time. High strike rates were seen in doctors with the highest workload and the least time available.

- a reluctance to record a PUN which would create an 'unwanted' DEN. Do not think of DENs when collecting PUNs. Defining DENs is a separate process that will be undertaken later. Do not feel inhibited when collecting PUNs – remember that the discovery page is personal and confidential to you. You do not have to address everything that you discover, but be honest with yourself while collecting PUNs.

You should aim for a strike rate above 10%. If it falls below this value you are either 'superdoc' or not looking hard enough. If it is over 50%, you are probably far too self-critical! Collect PUNs for a week, but if you haven't collected 10 PUNs by then, keep going until you have done so.

In Tables 3.1, 3.2, 3.3 and 3.4 below I list examples of the areas in which doctors discovered PUNs when we conducted the initial pilot study. The lists demonstrate the diversity of general practice. Some may cause you surprise that other doctors had difficulty in these areas, while you will identify with others. Problems with consultation skills were grossly under-reported. When things didn't go well, many doctors assumed that this was due to an attitudinal problem when in fact it was just a lack of skill in communication with particular groups (e.g. a teenager who brings a friend to see their GP, an anxious parent or someone with learning difficulties). You will no doubt identify with many of the attitudinal problems. It is surprising what irritates some doctors. One of them has a problem with smokers – that's a quarter of his patients he is already gunning for!

The doctor who is 'grumpy after 40 minutes of listening to a string of trivial complaints' needs to develop skills in ending a consultation! The poor doctor who is trying to 'reassure the hypochondriac' needs to recognise that such an approach is guaranteed to fail. And as for the one who is 'irritated by patient demand to discuss matters that only they think are important' – very patient centred! There is plenty of material for lively discussion with colleagues. The attitudes revealed in Table 3.4 are quite alarming. Some of them may be due to lack of training in consultation skills and how to use emotions that are experienced during consultations, but I suspect most of them are due to compassionate, caring doctors failing to perform because of high workloads and stress.

Table 3.1: Areas of discovery of PUNs in the pilot study: clinical knowledge

---

Antibiotic prescribing
Osteoporosis
Measles immunisation
Restless legs
Rashes
Hypertrophic obstructive cardiomyopathy (HOCM)
Back pain
Acne
Childhood migraine
Constipation in children
Breast cancer care
Persistent erections
Lumps on the tongue
Skin lesions
Dizzy spells
Development assessment
Helicobacter
Hypertension protocols
Stopping contraceptives prior to surgery

Continued

Table 3.1: *Continued*

Management of hip pain
Ring pessaries
Mastalgia
Frequency of blood glucose monitoring in diabetics
Rectal bleeding in a child
Vaginal discharge in the elderly
What to expect after a cataract operation on a 4-month-old
 child
Tennis elbow (how many injections and how often?)
Non-steroidal anti-inflammatory drugs and oesophageal
 stricture (are topical NSAIDs any good?)
Persistent arthralgia (Lyme's disease? salmonella?)
Chronic recurrent dizziness
Reliability of Rose–Waaler's test
Atrial fibrillation not controlled with digoxin
Use of clomiphene in general practice
Bladder problems in multiple sclerosis
Ankylosing spondylitis

The above list demonstrates the range of general practice – and we try to solve each one in 7 minutes without even knowing what might be coming in next! Genius or foolhardy?

Table 3.2: Areas of discovery of PUNs in the pilot study: non-clinical knowledge

---

The state benefit system
How long does it take for smear results to come back?
What drugs are illegal abroad?
The patient who wants a home delivery
Driving after a stroke

Continued

Table 3.2: *Continued*

Referral to surgical appliance department
Patient education books
Charges for signing an insurance form
Cost of over-the-counter drugs
Private hospital price list
Laser treatment for birthmarks
Do district nurses visit after a hysterectomy?
Filing a midstream urine result (filed and patient left untreated – what is the procedure?)
Local voluntary qualified counsellors
Practice flu jab protocol
Working part-time while on sick leave
Organisation/preparation for coil fitting
Which blood bottle should be used for HLA B27?

You won't find these answers in a textbook.

Table 3.3: Areas of discovery of PUNs in the pilot study: skills

Consultation skills
Elbow injection
Computer skills (multiple!)
Examining the nose
Reassuring the anxious mother
Introducing awareness of somatisation of affect
Removal of a mole
Wrist injection
Sigmoidoscopy

Deficiencies in consultation skills were missed and recorded as attitudinal problems.

Table 3.4: Areas of discovery of PUNs in the pilot study: attitudes

---

Irritation from DNAs (patients who did not attend) leading to poor performance with those who did attend.

Dealing with the following groups of patients who threatened one's desire to be caring and induced unpleasant feelings:

- the incurable
- smokers
- spongers
- urgent 'fitters in' when not ill
- 'while I'm here, doc'
- alcoholics
- drug addicts
- multiple problems; lists
- fat lazy 'thick' slobs

Stopping a patient talking too much

Not believing a patient's account of their alcohol intake

Intolerance of over-stated 'illness behaviour'

Coping with prospects of an 'inevitable suicide'

Grumpy after 40 minutes of listening to a string of trivial complaints

Reassuring the hypochondriac

Irritated by patient demand to discuss a matter that only they think is important

Disinterest in ME

Disinterest in a dull girl who is distressed about impending menarche

Intolerance of inadequate people who keep coming back despite 'knowing I can't help them further'

Intolerance of another middle-aged lady with multiple problems

---

'Attitudes' is an awful word. Having an attitude is always thought to be negative. How about using the terms 'beliefs' and 'values' instead? They sound much more positive.

Chapter 4

Examples of reflective learning

The following consultations are all real ones of my own, although the patients' names have been changed. They are here to show that reflecting on your consultations not only helps you discover your learning needs but that the process of reflection is educational in itself.

Practice organisation: the smear

The consultation

Enter Mrs Evans: 'The nurse said I had to see you for a smear, doctor, as she has taken it twice and both have been reported as "inadequate".' I suppressed my slight irritation that I was chosen, as I have partners who have a great interest in and excel at gynaecological procedures. (It takes all sorts!) Still, I've passed thousands of specula in my time, and last year's individual audit showed my success/failure rate to be no different to the others. Boosted by this memory, I ploughed on, still in buoyant mood. As no smear request form had already been completed for me, I rummaged in the drawers for a form. The patient sat politely (and presumably with some anxiety regarding her impending fate) while I continued to rummage. After a prolonged search in all of the drawers, I finally picked up the phone and rang the receptionist to ask for one. Awkward smiles ensued while I clasped the phone to my ear (... brrh ... brrh ... brrh ... brrh ... 'sorry' ... brrh ... brrh). I was thinking 'I don't care how hectic it is in reception – this is me, your doctor, calling – drop everything and get me a damn form'. I gave up, put the phone down. ('sorry' ...) and finally left the room to go and fetch the form myself. I returned with a pile of 50 forms, a sigh and an apology, which probably sounded more like 'you just can't get decent staff these days'. Anyway, we were back on track, I collected the details and Mrs Evans went behind the screen to prepare herself while I went to my trolley to organise ... quick check – gloves, speculum, slides, fixative, spatula ... pencil ... no pencil ... who has nicked my pencil? I learned years ago that writing on the slide

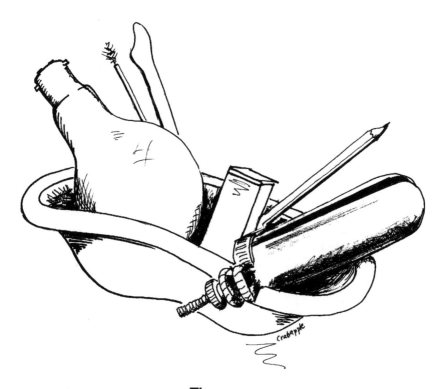

The smear.

afterwards was difficult, messy and is easy to forget. Should I start a search? I decided it was best to cope without the pencil and do it later. Concentrate on my patient ... rapport, reassurance, quick PV first ... ah ... difficult cervix to expose ... but I can handle it ... speculum in ... ah ... need the light ... right hand reaches out ... pull the light into position ... hit the switch ... no light! The bulb was missing! It was there on Friday – someone had nicked it. My professionalism, earlier challenged but since retrieved, was threatened again. Decision time. Is it gloves off, speculum out, leave patient starkers from the waist down, apologise profusely, go on hunt for light bulb and start all over again. Or do you do your best in the dark? You can probably guess what I did!

The PUN

The patient's needs were simple. She needed and deserved a slick, skilled, accurate cervical smear. I failed to meet her need on all counts.

Meeting the PUN

If I worked in hospital I could blame everyone else, but as a GP principal I am director of a small business and its efficiency is down to me. We have been looking at PUNs in our practice for several years now, and these types of problems had been uncovered before and, I thought, had been successfully tackled. I knew that the duty receptionist was meant to check the forms and the practice nurse was responsible for checking the trolleys, but who should check the light bulbs? The commonest way of dealing with these kinds of problems is to rant at the practice manager, who can then in turn rant at the staff. This approach invariably upsets everyone, nothing changes, and we can do the same thing all over again next week. We do have a system for checking consulting-rooms that usually works well, but if only one receptionist is off sick, it is impossible for the others to get away from the desk to check the rooms. Of course, if I had bothered to notice that we were short-staffed I would simply have fetched the forms without attempting to ring reception first, and I would have been a lot less irritated as a result. As for the pencil, it was on the trolley all the time – I just couldn't see it. The smear result has just come back 'negative' with transition zone (TZ) sampling. I never did discover what happened to my light bulb, but it goes to show that if you can't always shed light on a problem, then feeling your way in the dark can still produce results – a bit like general practice really!

Box 4.1: Main learning points

- Develop structures with your staff to make your life easier.
- Be aware that receptionists have a difficult job to do as well.
- Don't automatically blame everyone else when things go wrong (it could possibly be no one's fault).
- Accept that however well prepared you are, things will still go wrong sometimes.

Clinical knowledge: peanut allergy

The consultation

The computer told me that my next patient was an 8-year-old boy, but only his mother came in. 'I've come to get the results of the blood tests,' she said. I didn't know the patient or the history, so I attempted three things at once – to be welcoming and offer a seat, size up the patient (a sort of body language psychosocial history!) and scroll through the computer notes to grasp what it was all about. The mother appeared to be a pleasant sensible woman with a straightforward request. The computer told me that consultations had occurred with three different doctors, the last doctor had performed some RAST tests, and it was these results that we were after. The patient's mother and I looked at the screen together. 'I didn't ask for Brazil nuts,' she said. On the screen was a list of different types of nut with a number next to each one. They were all labelled 0 except for 'peanut', which was labelled 2. 'They're all 0 except peanuts, which are 2', I said hopefully. 'What does 2 mean?,' she asked. Good question, I thought. 'Well, you can score from 0 to 6, so 2 is worse than 1 but nowhere near as bad as 6,' I heard myself saying. Remembering previous disasters, and realising what a prat I must have sounded, I quickly came clean. I thought, 'Why didn't you come and see the clever dick who requested the investigation in the first place?', but I said 'to be honest, I don't know very much about allergies; I'm afraid you've come to the wrong doctor as I really don't have the knowledge to help you.' I smiled and hoped she might say 'Oh well, never mind, sorry to have wasted your time, I should have come back to Dr Smith, after

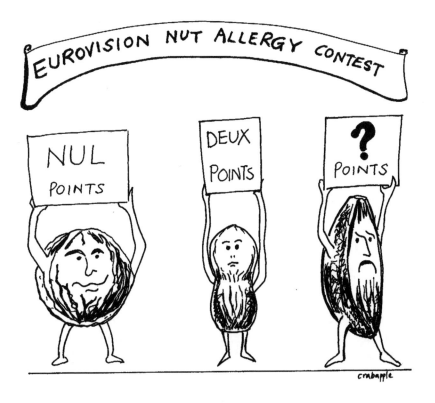

'Wal and Pea have declared, but there seems to be a problem
with Brazil ...'

all it was he who requested the test.' However, she didn't say that and she didn't smile – I sensed that she was not impressed by my candour. She didn't leave, and instead she insisted on more questions. I sensed that she didn't want a wasted journey and she felt that if she pushed me hard enough I might still come up with some answers. I found myself explaining that the more sensitive you are to something, the more IgE you make in response to it, and it was good news that her son was only allergic to peanuts. 'Not at all', she said, 'he may be very allergic to Brazil nuts but I've never given him any, so he has not had the opportunity to make any IgE.' I hadn't thought of that. She finally left with a resolve to come back and see someone who knew what they were talking about.

The PUN

This patient expressed a clear need for interpretation of the test results, and I failed to meet it. Reflecting on the consultation, I realised all the other needs that might have been behind her failure to return my smile. I imagined what it must be like to have a small child with a serious nut allergy. No flying round Sainsbury's after work, but instead a meticulous obsessive study of all food labels, watching everything they eat, risking them going to children's parties or being offered snacks by friends at school, and carrying adrenaline and wondering whether to give it. There were clearly enormous needs crying out for support.

Meeting the PUN

1 *Define a personal DEN.* I don't have the time or the interest to be an expert, but as a generalist I do need to know more. I shall start by searching the Internet, and will

also give the librarian a ring to see if she can come up with a helpful review article.

2 *Delegation.* I don't think there is a local expert to refer to, but there might be. I shall telephone my friendly paediatrician and ask her for advice. There's bound to be a nut allergy support group – my manager will track it down for me, and perhaps come up with some useful leaflets.

3 *Practice organisation.* I shall discuss this case with my partners and practice nurses, particularly the individual who requested the RAST tests! There are several issues to explore. What in-house knowledge do we already have? Why has this patient 'doctor-hopped'? Was there difficulty in getting appointments? Do my partners want to learn with me? Is there an interest in exploring this together or is this one down to me alone?

Just one consultation has stimulated me to add agenda to my personal learning portfolio, to communicate with secondary care services and to explore issues within the practice. If I happened to have attended a lecture from an immunologist on RAST tests before the consultation, my embarrassment during the consultation would have been less, but learning with PUNs and DENs actually stimulates change.

Attitudes: the heartsink patient

The consultation

Mrs Glossop comes to see you. 'I've come to have my blood pressure taken – you haven't taken it for ages.' While she takes off a few layers, you rummage in a drawer for the large cuff that might just reach round her arm. You know Mrs Glossop – in fact you hate Mrs Glossop. You have found her to be demanding, rude, ungrateful and impossible to satisfy. Her blood pressure is 200/110 and she is already on two drugs to control it. You are about to ask whether she remembers to take her tablets when you recall asking her once before – it didn't go down well! Your aim now is to get her out of the consulting-room as quickly as possible and to adopt the strategy of saying nothing, and certainly not asking any questions. You add a drug to her long list, print it out, tell her that she needs another pill for her blood pressure and hand it over with all of the body language you can muster that says 'goodbye'. Dream on! 'You've given me these pills before and they gave me terrible indigestion – it should all be on the computer. And don't give me those red ones that gave me a headache, either.' You feel trapped, but she changes the subject and starts on about your practice nurse knowing nothing about diabetes and how she would starve to death on the diet she advised. Her voice drones on. You stopped listening ages ago, but you make a final effort: 'What we will do, Mrs Glossop, is leave your treatment as it is for now, but check your blood pressure again in a couple of weeks.' She finally leaves, only to return in two weeks' time and go through it all again.

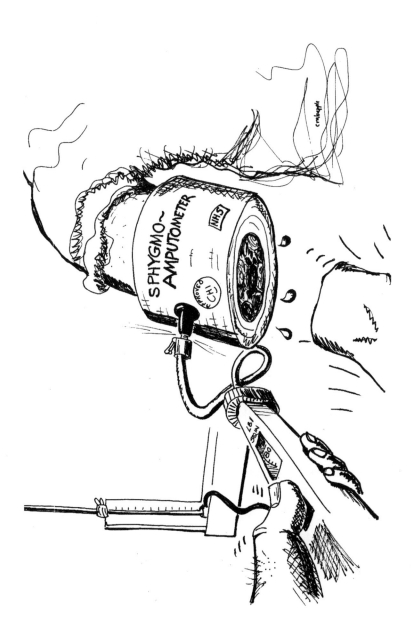

'Just pop your arm in here.'

Deciphering wants and needs

Heartsink patients can become quite an issue with new doctors, and they provide ideal material to bring to a small group. It is all very well to offload and share the burden, but there are strategies to help you solve the problem. Focusing on the details of what was said or inferred by either party often identifies what is really going on, and the dysfunction is then understood. After describing the case to the group, try one of the following methods.

- *Patient's wants*: to be a patient, receive attention, make you feel inadequate.

- *Doctor's wants*: for Mrs Glossop to go away and never return, or to see someone else, or at least to listen to advice, show some respect and do something to help herself.

- *Patient's needs* (Be brave here, use your common sense or instinct): what do you really know about Mrs Glossop? Did you know about her unhappy marriage and abusive husband? Did you know that she had two stillbirths and has one daughter who doesn't keep in touch with her because of her abusive father? Did you know how depressed and lonely she is? She needs to come to terms with her unhappy marriage and adopt a strategy to regain her daughter.

- *Doctor's needs*: to be able to recognise and control any emotions that are generated, and to use consultation skills, such as open questions, to focus on the real issues. Once the real problem has been identified and shared, the doctor may choose to develop the skills necessary to address the problem, or they may elect to refer the patient to someone who already has those skills.

Exploring the doctor's feelings

Feelings can be voiced in a small, supportive, professionally led group, but care must be taken. A useful model is that of persecutor–victim–rescuer. Many doctors are natural rescuers, but natural victims are by no means rare. Victims have an inner need to feel overpowered or threatened, and therefore avoid escaping heartsinks – some doctors even collect them.

Box 4.2: Main learning points for dealing with heartsink patients

- Recognise your own emotions, understand where they come from and use them to your advantage.
- Differentiate between the patient's wants and needs.
- Use your consultation skills to focus on the real needs.
- Share heartsinks and difficult consultations with colleagues – you are not alone!

Team working: drug budget

The consultation

It was always a pleasure to see Kate. I had known her since she was a teenager. Life had never been easy for her, and I had had the privilege of helping her through many a hard time. I think she valued our relationship and the personal care that I provided. I knew her extended family and her husband well. They were both employed, poorly paid, not on benefit and paid taxes. She brought a bundle of papers and came straight to the point. 'Martin and I have finally saved enough money to try again for IVF. We would both be so grateful if you would prescribe the drugs for us again.' It was nearly three years now since their first failed attempt. I smiled and said that I would be more than happy to help. I set about producing the prescription, said that I would administer injections as and when required, and handed over about £800 worth of drugs. Kate left happy with her needs well met.

The PUN

Here is a consultation with no PUN. My patient's needs were fully met. She was in need and I was in a position to help. If I had kept this consultation to myself, that would be the end of the story.

The DEN

Later that day, while I was signing my prescriptions my senior partner walked by and I casually mentioned that I had spent £800 of our drug budget on one patient. He said nothing.

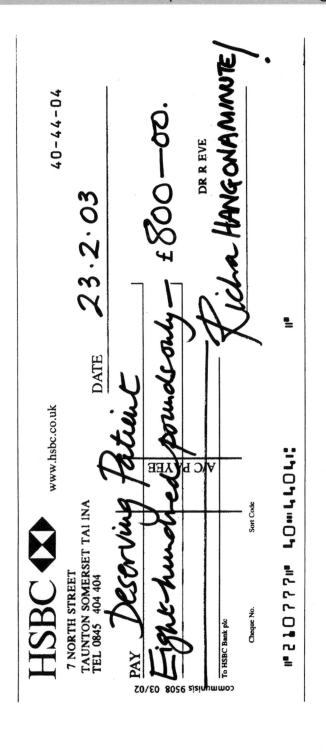

Later, at the end of a lunchtime meeting, he did have things to say. David is our prescribing lead. He has introduced effective control systems into our practice and successfully made us all much more aware of cost-effective prescribing. Only the day before he had introduced a way to reduce our spending. He had highlighted the fact that there were patients on ACE inhibitors such as ramipril 2.5 mg twice a day. If we changed all of these to 5 mg once a day we could save £2000 – sensible cost-effective prescribing. On a whim I had thrown away half his savings. I could see his frustration.

What followed was the type of meeting that I try to avoid. It may have been disorganised, but it was an opportunity to let off steam. First there was, 'The budget is too small. Our energies should be directed towards enlarging the budget. Any attempts to keep within the budget imply that we accept it.' And then, 'I am my patient's advocate. I will continue to do what I think is best for my patient. The drug bill is not my problem.' Alternatively, 'We must accept the reality of the situation. Primary care is budgeted and we must accept responsibility for staying in budget' or 'if we don't make choices they will be made for us by politicians, and who knows our patients' priorities best?', and worst of all, 'if you don't keep in budget, the staff budget will be reduced and people will lose their jobs'. Confronted with 'control your prescribing or sack the counsellor', I could only feel anger. We ended by discussing the stupidity of GPs being given two contradictory messages – on the one hand to be more aggressive in their treatment of hypertension and cholesterol in order to save lives, and on the other hand to reduce their spending on drugs (all this while the price of drugs is rising!). I expect we all felt confused, disempowered, frustrated and angry by the end of the meeting.

I've since spoken to a friend in another practice. He admitted that they have an agreed practice policy on not prescribing infertility drugs. They talk of a postcode lottery! It seems that, at the moment, the particular doctor whom you see within our practice determines whether you will receive infertility drugs. Within the town it depends on which practice you register with. Do we need a practice protocol? Do we need a primary care group-based protocol? Do we need a countywide directive? Do we not need a nationwide Government directive?

My learning needs

There is no problem with my knowledge or prescribing skills. It is my 'attitude' that needs to be developed. The awful truth is that I am prepared to deny my patient the infertility drugs as long as *it's not my fault*. I can't function as an effective GP if I am not my patient's advocate. Government policy is to restrict resources (i.e. control costs) in a way that *is not their fault*. For a while, until I am forced to rethink, I have decided to adopt the ostrich strategy. I am not going to write to my primary care trust, lobby my MP or write to Tony Blair. I am going to keep my head down and quietly continue doing what I think is right and in my patient's best interest. I shall remain my own judge as to whether I am responsible with regard to my spending of NHS resources. If and when 'authority' wishes to challenge my activity, I shall defend myself. As I see it, I am first and foremost accountable to my patients, myself and my profession – a view that I fear will soon be thought old-fashioned.

Non-clinical knowledge

It is surprising how often things go wrong or the patient's needs are left unmet because of a lack of simple non-clinical knowledge. From not knowing how to use the computer, find a form or make an appropriate referral, a consultation can easily become dysfunctional. Non-clinical knowledge can easily affect your management.

Your clinical judgement may indicate a referral to the pain clinic, but if you knew that the waiting-list to be seen was over a year, then you would probably come up with an alternative strategy. The threshold for referral depends on your knowledge of the local situation. If you had an effective responsive multidisciplinary family therapy unit, then your threshold for referring possible attention deficit hyperactivity disorder would be much lower. The way in which you manage drug abuse depends on the availability of an effective local support programme. A few years ago, before we had a physiotherapist in the practice, I almost gave up referring any patients to physiotherapy services, not because of any doubts about the quality of care or long waiting-lists, but simply because the effort of getting there outweighed any possible benefit from the treatment. Parking was impossible, cut-throat and stressful, and when one did finally manage to park, if one could walk that far to the department one probably didn't need the treatment anyway! To be effective in meeting your patients' needs, you require a mass of knowledge concerning the quantity, quality and availability of secondary and support services.

The consultation

I was expecting Mr James, but Mrs James came alone wanting to discuss her husband. She had a large trolley with her and she took out several folders of paper work, all of which related to her husband's care. They are an elderly couple with a significant number of problems, but they struggle on independently. They are intelligent and resourceful and have a lovely flat, but I confess to having grown weary of listening to tales of woe and misery. I probably wasn't listening carefully enough but it transpired that they both received an Attendance Allowance for looking after each other, and Mrs James now wanted me to complete a DS1500 for her husband so that his application for the higher rate of allowance could go through 'fast track'. He was recently diagnosed with a slow-growing squamous-cell carcinoma of the anus and was going to receive some radiotherapy. I explained that we didn't consider this problem to be terminal or his demise to be imminent, so the special rules did not apply. Mrs James persisted and pointed out that although I was meant to expect death within 6 months it couldn't possibly be guaranteed, and that this therefore gave leeway for me to sign. Of course I relented I went and found a DS1500, completed it and handed it over. In my mind we had a deal – I'll sign this if you will go away now. No such luck! She obviously felt that she had caught me at a weak moment, and she ploughed on with her next request, which was for a wheelchair for herself. I didn't even bother to point out that her legs seemed to work OK and that she didn't even use a stick, but I went in with what I thought would be a winner – 'but your husband is far too unwell to push a wheelchair'. She swiftly replied 'Oh no doctor, I mean an electric one to use when out shopping.' I waffled (... we could discuss this some other time ... etc.) and resorted to one of my firmer 'end of consultation' manoeuvres by getting up and holding the door open for her to leave.

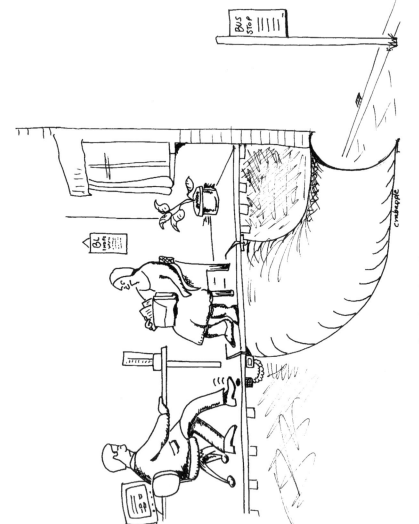

Getting rid of Mrs James.

I share this consultation as an example demonstrating my lack of non-clinical knowledge in not knowing how to acquire a wheelchair, but perhaps the consultation is really telling me to acquire the skills in how not to acquire one! My inability to define and focus on Mrs James' true needs allowed a dysfunctional consultation to take place in which I endeavoured to comply with her 'wants', in the hope that she would then go away.

There was a time when we had a local wheelchair clinic. A quick referral note was required and the experts then assessed the needs and passed the patient and their details on to the Wheelchair Centre at Exeter. Now I think I have to refer directly and fill in some dreadful form with questions that I don't understand. I have identified a DEN and will need to explore whether I can delegate it somewhere, otherwise I will have to find space in my brain for even more knowledge.

Telephone consultations

The identification of PUNs is not limited to the consulting-room. A two-minute phone call got me thinking.

The consultation

I was manning the phone at our local out-of-hours co-op, and it was pretty busy. A call came through from a smart-sounding woman: 'I've got cystitis again and could you leave out some antibiotics?' It was about 9 p.m. My initial thoughts were that the chemists were now shut (we would need our emergency supply) and the word 'again' concerned me. The quickest solution would be to check that she wasn't allergic to trimethoprim, leave out six tablets for her to collect and move on to the next call. Instead I enquired about the symptoms that led her to believe she had cystitis, and I asked how frequent a problem it was. I sensed in her voice a slight irritation that I was not prepared just to accept her own diagnosis and treatment plan. My judgement was that this was not something best managed with a 'quick fix', and that it would be more appropriate for her to present during normal working hours to her own GP with a urine sample. I explained that we needed to establish whether her 'recurrent cystitis' was truly infective, and that a midstream urine specimen should be collected before starting any antibiotics. I advised her to drink plenty of fluids in the mean time. I also thought that she was using the out-of-hours service as a convenience and that her problem did not merit emergency attention, although I did not share this thought with her. A few days later, the co-op manager sent me a copy of this patient's letter of complaint. She had found my

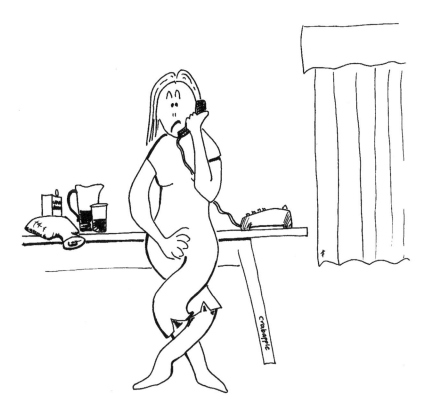

'Drink plenty of water, and call me in the morning.'

attitude patronising and was particularly annoyed that she had to take time off work the next day, and that she had to waste her own and her GP's time. It was all quite unnecessary and all my fault (a view that would have been enhanced if her GP had given her a ten-second consultation and antibiotics with no exploration).

The patient's wants

So what can be learned from this? Here was a busy intelligent woman who knew just what she wanted. She was a consumer of a public service in Blair's Britain, expecting a 'quick fix' and instant access. Was her demand unreasonable? If my wife was in her position, she certainly wouldn't be taking time off work to see her GP. She would expect me to hand over the antibiotics. In this busy modern world it does seem that I was unreasonable not to meet her demands.

The patient's needs

Were the patient's 'needs' exactly the same as her 'wants'? I questioned this, and that is why I was in trouble. Something made me think that there was more to it. Was it just that I felt she should concentrate more on her health than on her diary? Didn't she need a proper diagnosis? Was it really a recurrent infection or was it honeymoon cystitis? Did she need to sit down with her GP and explore why this was happening, or take preventative measures? Was her lifestyle relevant? Were there hidden fears to be explored? (If she was reading this, I can imagine her saying 'you can't even get a urinary tract infection treated without a full psychosexual social history!' – she would have a point.)

The doctor's wants

I think that I wanted to be helpful, but as far as she was concerned I was difficult. Was I really delaying her treatment so that what I perceived to be her true 'needs' could be met properly? What she regarded as a waste of her own and her GP's time I saw as an opportunity for better care. Or was it the case that what I really wanted was to express the 'baggage' that I carried? I was annoyed that she had made her own diagnosis and treatment plan. She didn't want a doctor – she wanted an antibiotic. She was abusing the out-of-hours system. Urinary tract infections are not emergencies. It was her convenience, not her health, that was her priority. If we give in to this 24-hour consumer demand approach, the out-of-hours service will not be able to cope. Someone must make a stand. What I really wanted to do was to tell her that her problem was not an emergency and that she was wasting my time, which would be better spent on those who were really ill.

The DENs

So what educational needs have I discovered from this episode? How bad is cystitis? Does it merit out-of-hours treatment?

I discussed this episode with a female doctor who told me from personal experience that dysuria is real agony, and that the symptoms can start to improve within a few hours of swallowing the first antibiotic tablet. I could tell that she felt that I had been unkind. However, the *NHS Direct Healthcare Guide* advises self-care and also states 'Drink plenty of fluids and take paracetamol. A covered hot-water bottle on your tummy also helps. If there is no improvement after two days, call NHS Direct.' I am sure that the silent majority suffer quietly at home and don't want to trouble the doctor out of hours. The informed consumer expects more. If we provide out-of-hours treatment to one patient, then shouldn't we be advertising to the others 'don't suffer in silence – we provide a 24-hour get-started-on-antibiotic-service'?

Personal care or convenience?

Do you wish to see any doctor now or wait to see your own doctor? We have two populations out there – those who value personal care and will wait for it, and the consumers who want quick access to any doctor. It seems that we will need to adapt to meet the needs of both. We will need to learn how to maximise care and minimise risk in providing a one-stop service.

Consistency in out-of-hours care

Having spoken to many colleagues, their 'baggage' seems to fit into one of two main categories. One group feels that primary care was not set up or funded to provide 24-hour routine care. If we do not make an effort to resist consumer demand to provide it, personal care will be lost and the out-of-hours service will collapse. Doctors in this group feel that they have a duty to remind patients that the out-of-hours service is emergency only. The other group is simply working an out-of-hours shift. They will see anyone who wants to see them, and they will avoid any confrontation. The aim is to get through the shift with minimal exposure to personal criticism or risk of complaint. When their shift is over, it is no longer their problem – rather like working in Accident and Emergency.

At the moment, our patients/clients/consumers run a lottery for non-emergency care out of hours depending on which doctor is on duty, what mood they are in and how busy they are. This situation is not ideal, but I think it is still better than trying to put together a consensus protocol. Where would be the fun in that?

Bringing 'baggage' to the consultation

The consultation

I checked the notes on the computer before my next patient arrived. He had joined the list about eight weeks ago. In that time he had had five 'urgent slot' consultations, each with a different doctor (two locums, the retainee and two partners). He was officially registered with me. On each occasion he had left with a sick note for either one or two weeks saying 'depression'. He was a drug user. I felt that it was time for this issue to be addressed. Either he should receive a long-term sick note (to stop him coming back every week for another one) and an appropriate referral, or else I would tell him that I did not consider him to be 'sick' and that he should make himself available for work. It was decision time. He shuffled in and sat down. 'I've come for my sick note.' If it is possible to walk, sit and speak disrespectfully, he managed it. 'What is the nature of your illness?,' I enquired. He looked confused. 'What have doctors been writing on your sick note?,' I tried. 'It doesn't matter – I use drugs, I need the giro' was the gist of his reply. Without making much of an assessment I felt that I didn't like this man, and I found him rude, aggressive and demanding. I decided that he was not going to get a sick note from me. He grew more angry and I refused to oblige. We reached a silent impasse. I felt nervous and stood up to walk round him to the door so that I could show him out or make my escape. Suddenly he leapt up, blocked my path, grabbed me by my shirt and tie just below my neck and pushed me up against the wall. I sensed that he wasn't going to leave without a sick note! My left hand was within inches of the panic button. I didn't use it, as I felt that the sudden noise would be the signal for him to put a fist in my face. Instead I submitted. I gave him a sick note for one week marked 'aggression'. He grabbed it and left without reading it.

The PUN

It was quite clear what the patient 'wanted' – a sick note. He wanted the cheque either to buy drugs or to pay off someone who was threatening him. What were his real 'needs'? I didn't get very far in assessing them, but I suppose he needed a productive relationship with a professional carer. He needed to trust someone. He needed to realise that a GP could have more to offer than a sick note. And perhaps he needed to learn some slightly more subtle communication skills!

The DEN

I learned a lot from this encounter. When colleagues had been frightened by violent patients I was sympathetic but in the back of my mind I always wondered whether they could have handled these incidents better. In 20 years of general practice this was the only time I had been attacked. I thought that I would always be able to manipulate my way out of direct confrontation. Now I had learned that I wasn't special and that I was as vulnerable as anyone else.

I had never realised how upsetting it is to be attacked. After the patient had left I went and sat with the receptionists. I felt quite weak at the knees and my heart was racing. It took a good ten minutes and a cup of tea before I felt that I could continue with the surgery. From now on when my partners, nurses or receptionists tell me that they feel frightened or threatened by a patient, I shall really understand and be very supportive.

I learned the hard way the folly of prejudging a patient.

Essentially I had decided that I wasn't going to give him a sick note before he even came into the room, and he had decided that he would not be leaving without one. Two entrenched positions inevitably led to confrontation. It is a shame that we didn't catch it on video. I wonder if I was gunning for this guy right from the start. I was in an assertive mood that day and clever-dick Eve was going to get the matter sorted where everyone else had avoided the issue. I had brought 'baggage' to the consultation.

I had allowed my assertive mood, prejudice and prejudgement to block my ability to apply my consultation skills effectively. Needless to say, the patient was thrown off the list and I have not seen him since. Sometimes I reflect on this poor disturbed disadvantaged young man who was desperate for his giro, and at other times I think of this nasty thug and how I would like to punch him in the eye.

Arthur's dilemma

The consultation

I've known Arthur for 15 years. A few years ago his wife was ill. Her sister moved in to look after them both. His wife died, and her sister stayed on to look after him. Within weeks she died as well. All alone and unable even to learn how to boil an egg, Arthur sold up and moved into a residential home. He's been the fittest resident ever since. He is 91 years old now and still going strong – taking pills for prostate and hypertension, pretty deaf, mobile enough to pace himself down to the surgery, but chronically depressed, biding his time until he goes to join his wife. Last week, on his monthly visit to see me, I found him in atrial fibrillation, with no complaints and no signs of failure. Blood tests and ECG were arranged, and here he was back to see me. Carefully and slowly (and loudly) I explained the choice in front of him – aspirin or warfarin. I probably summed up with 'reduction of stroke risk is 50% with aspirin and 80% with warfarin. What do you want to do?' He paused and looked at me. 'You're my doctor, you decide.' It was rather like 'what's the point in having a dog and barking yourself?'. He had the intellectual ability to address the problem, but as far as he was concerned he would trust my decision totally. He wanted to put his life in my hands!

The PUN

Arthur's *wants* are pretty clear. The cook feeds him, the cleaner cleans, the optician provides appropriate glasses, the

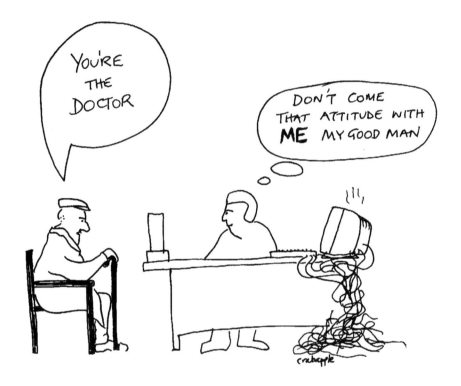

Arthur.

accountant checks his finances, the stockbroker looks after his investments and the doctor does his health. He wants whatever is in his best interests, and he expects me to deliver it without bothering him.

What are Arthur's *needs*? The smart answer is that he needs to realise that he must take responsibility for his own health, and therefore I should now move the consultation on towards meeting that need. I should decline to absolve him of responsibility. A common problem with registrars and new GPs is that they take on patients' major problems and then get in a mess as they transfer the problem on to themselves, rather than remembering that they are there to help the patient with their problem, not to take it on themselves. As a teacher, if a colleague brought me this dilemma I would easily give them the smart answer. But this time I feel stuck. Who am I to decide Arthur's needs? Perhaps his wants are his needs. He is delegating his health to me. His needs seem to be a perfectly reasonable delegation of responsibility to me. After all, I am the doctor.

The DEN

I seem to be stuck, unable to decide whether Arthur's need is to accept responsibility for his own health or to delegate that responsibility to me. I like Arthur – he is a friend and I respect him. He also respects me and I want to do my best for him. I understand him. His request is alien to my training and professionalism, but emotionally I want to meet his expectation and take on the responsibility. I thought of sharing my problem with a more senior colleague, but I could already visualise his wry smile as he told me that it didn't really matter what I did and that I was fussing over nothing. Arthur may or may not take prescribed treatment. He may die this year, next year or 10 years from now. He was telling me that he didn't really care. If it was important to him, he wouldn't be trusting me with a decision! That was it! Arthur didn't care and so the decision was not the big conflict I had made for myself. The decision between aspirin and warfarin was not important.

So what have I learned from this consultation? By a process of personal reflection I feel that I have resolved the issue. I have learned that work and more work without time for reflection is of poor quality. I have learned that there is more to good medicine than reading guidelines, research papers and risk assessment. I have learned that it is OK to allow your emotions to contribute in consultations with patients, but most of all, if you are going to get it right you must find time for reflection.

And if you are wondering whether Arthur got warfarin or aspirin, I am not going to tell you, because taking everything into consideration, it doesn't really matter!

PUNs and computers

This week I managed to find a PUN for every consultation in the afternoon surgery. It started badly and got progressively worse. We had to shut down the computer system for the afternoon in order to add an upgrade. We were not too daunted by this because we had shut down for two full days previously. On that occasion we were highly organised and everything went according to plan. We downloaded all of the booked appointments on to our laptops, and all of the staff and patients were prepared.

The consultation

I rolled up confidently, attached my laptop to the printer and the receptionist came in with a small collection of messages. Mrs Davies wanted to discuss her blood results. A psychiatric patient said that she had lost her prescription and was waiting in reception for another. Could I ring a GP in Wales who had one of our patients with him requesting a methadone script? And could I instantly fill in Mr Brown's form outlining his medication, as he was waiting for it and going into hospital in the morning? These were all needs I couldn't meet. I left the work to my receptionist. Tell Mrs Davies that I will ring her tomorrow. Tell the Welsh GP that I can't help until tomorrow. Tell Mr Brown to go without his form and dig out a copy of his repeat prescription, and I will see the psychiatric patient now to resolve something. Inevitably that was not straightforward, and I finally started surgery late. The first patient arrived and I tried to be attentive, but I realise that most of the time I played with my laptop, trying to review her history. I can't even remember what the consultation was about, but I know that she needed a prescription for something and a repeat of her 'usual'. Next disaster – no response from the printer. I wasted much time checking cables and power supplies and fiddling with buttons before I noticed that the laptop had informed me that there was 'no printing module available'. I was going to have to write out all of the scripts by hand, but at least I had a list of medication in front of me. Until the next patient, that is! Mrs James wanted her husband's repeat medication while she was there. You would think it would be easy to explain that since neither of us knew what the drugs were, she would have to wait and request the prescription in the normal way tomorrow. She seemed to take this as a personal insult. It would cause her great inconvenience. Didn't I know what it was like to have a disabled husband? Then followed a tirade about the inefficiency of our practice, from the failings of our repeat script system to the difficulties of getting appointments and the attitude of our staff. Congratulations to Mrs James, for she had managed to turn a reasonably caring doctor into an uncaring irritable wild animal. From now on all patients were seen as the enemy. For the rest of the surgery I failed to identify patients' met or unmet needs. I no longer cared what their needs were. It was my needs that mattered – turn them over, get them out and go home.

The patient's wants and needs

Normally I would have handled Mrs James quite easily. I might even have explored what was underlying her anger, and I certainly would not have taken it personally. In fact, I missed an opportunity to discover her true needs, uncover her depression and offer the services of those who support

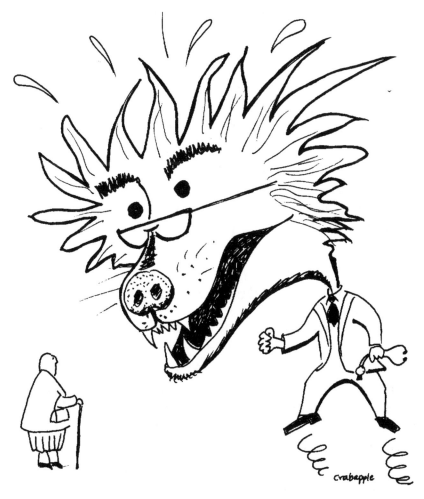

'I just wanted my pills, Doctor.'

carers. So what went wrong? It was not having the computer. *A GP without a database is like a surgeon without a knife.* The quality and efficiency of our service now depends on computers. Without instant access to data we are unable to cope.

Most of the problems confronting me related to patient wants or demands. Because of computer technology we found it easy to meet those demands, and patients have now become used to getting an immediate response. We have raised patient expectations, and this can only cause trouble. If you expect very little, you are easily satisfied. If you expect a lot, dissatisfaction is inevitable. All of the problems that were presented for me to solve before I started surgery weren't real needs, but rather they were wants engendered by the increase in expectation.

The doctor's educational needs

So what have I learned? What do I need to learn or change? Is there material for my personal development plan or for my practice to learn? How can three hours without the computer cause so much trouble? I can cope with a medical emergency just as well with or without a computer. It seems that we only ran into trouble because we tried so hard. We loaded up our laptops, and the receptionists had to deal with every individual who phoned up or walked in. At our next practice meeting I shall suggest a new approach. Block out all patient contacts except emergencies. Lock the surgery doors and put up a notice explaining that we are closed and a phone number for emergencies. Put the following message on an answerphone: 'The surgery is closed this afternoon for a computer upgrade. Please leave all routine enquiries, appointments and repeat prescriptions until tomorrow. If you have an emergency, please ring ...' The computer has become central to all patient demands, and attempts to continue operating result in dissatisfied customers. Of course, the answerphone message could cause much irritation and dissatisfaction, but then I won't know because I'm not available!

Chapter 5

Research to reality

By reflecting on what we do and discovering PUNs, we soon collect a number of DENs that we now want to fulfil. Medicine develops at an incredible pace. Not only do we have new ways of managing disease and new drugs, but we even have new diseases. I remember when heartburn and the menopause were symptoms of life. We now have gastro-oesophageal reflux disease (GORD) and a billion pound industry in hormone replacement therapy. A cynic might think that drug companies not only find new drugs for diseases, but are even inventing the diseases for their drugs! I recently found PUNs in both of these areas. A 40-year-old man had been told by the specialist that he must take a proton-pump inhibitor 'for life'. The drug upset him and he wanted to know what risk he was taking if he just took the tablets occasionally. A recent media scare had alarmed a woman on continuous combined hormone replacement therapy, and she wanted to know about her risks. Not only did these patients want knowledge – they also wanted my opinion. In order to help these patients I needed more knowledge.

Evidence-based medicine (EBM) is there to help me. If a general physician wishes to keep abreast of their field, they will need to get to grips with 19 original articles per day for 365 days a year. Of these, only 2% will pass quality clinical and scientific criteria. Which ones are they? I don't have time for that! Meta-analysis might be helpful, but the outcome simply depends on which papers they select for inclusion. I

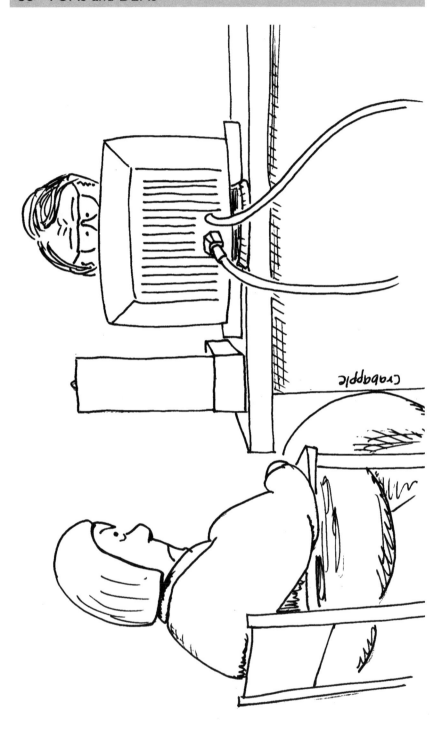

could obtain some review articles, and a good local librarian should be able to find me these. Or best of all, I could refer to the Cochrane Database of Systematic Reviews in the hope that they have actually covered the area in which I am interested. These days we can get answers in a language that is easier to understand, such as number needed to treat (NNT). I like to write to my local specialist in the area and ask them what best evidence is telling us at the moment. Without too much effort I can obtain a manageable amount of written evidence. In this way I can increase my knowledge and gain awareness of what research has to say on the matter.

EBM has given me information on statistical significance. It tells me what happened to specific trial populations. To get into a trial as a patient you often have to be a bit of a freak – on no other medication, with no other diseases, belonging to a restricted age group and totally compliant with taking medication and follow-up. I will have to consider how relevant this evidence is to my own practice population and circumstances. In the example of GORD, how much of the evidence is based on trials funded by drug companies? There may be a recommended best practice, but in my practice many things may influence what I actually do. Does my local hospital buy in an expensive proton-pump inhibitor (PPI) at bulk discount? Does my primary care trust have guidance on cost-effective PPI prescribing? Does it have a formulary? Does my practice have a formulary? Will changing to best practice destroy my drug budget? Will I need more endoscopies? Is there direct access to endoscopy? Is the waiting-list so long that you can't get them? In practice I may have to compromise my aspirations for 'best practice' and settle for something more realistic. We are turning a statistical significance into a clinical one.

Having looked at the research and seen how it may be possible to bring change into practice, there is still much to do.

$$\text{Effort} = \text{desire} \times \text{expectation} \qquad \text{(vroom)}$$

The amount of effort that I put into something is a combination of my desire to do it and my expectation that it will be worthwhile or successful. My desire to win the lottery is enormous, but my expectation of winning is so low that I don't even bother to buy a ticket! I must believe that a new treatment will bring real benefit. The whole process of bringing about change is complicated, and there is no shortage of 'change consultants' in industry. Before I will change my practice I have to feel uncomfortable with my present practice. The evidence that 'Septrin' was bad and trimethoprim was good was long established before I could actually bring myself to write a longer word, and only half the drug, on a prescription pad. We now find that beta-blockers don't cause heart failure but that we should be using them to treat it. Experts must understand that there is more to introducing change than publishing a research paper, and they must be patient when we are slow to respond.

Once we are uncomfortable with present practice, we will still resist change unless there is a mechanism in place to help us to make that change. Even the simplest changes are not easy. According to best practice, sustained-release nifedipine and diltiazem should not be generic prescriptions – and most of ours were. We should choose one manufacturer and stick to them. A simple change like this involved the practice manager, the local pharmacist, practice nurses and receptionists as well as all of the partners agreeing on which drug to choose. Administrative, organisational and IT skills were all needed. A dysfunctional organisation could not even start to make a simple change like this. Modern general practice is dependent on quality management, organisation and teamwork.

I think I have nearly cracked it now – I know what is best practice, I believe in it and I want to change. I have created an environment in my practice that can adapt to change and implement mechanisms for change. I have focused on teambuilding and communications. All that is left is to make that change in the consulting-room ... and in walks Mrs Glossop.

I have brought statistical significance down to clinical significance, and now I have to translate that into personal significance in the one-to-one consultation. The whole range of competencies required of a good doctor, as described in Chapter 1, now comes into play. Medical science informs us about what is best practice, but what is best practice for Mrs Glossop, Mrs James or Arthur?

Are we here to inflict treatment and health on patients in order to improve statistics on population morbidity and mortality, or should we use our medical knowledge and best practice to offer the best possible care to an individual? Historically, as GPs we have only been there to help individuals and to be their advocate, but now we also have responsibility for the health of populations.

Experts view risk as a quantifiable statistic and assume that everyone wants the lowest risk. This is to assume that anyone with any sense, when they go to the races, must put their money on the favourite. Well, life isn't like that. You pick your horse for all sorts of reasons – you're a friend of the owner, you know the jockey, pretty colours, pretty horse, it looks fit on the day, you feel lucky, lucky number, etc. Life is not a statistic, and people do not behave according to reason or logic. Risk taking is a very complex part of human nature.

A paper published in the *British Medical Journal* explored a system which involved patients in a decision-making process with regard to whether or not they wanted to take warfarin to treat atrial fibrillation.[1] It was found that when patients made their own informed risk assessment it did not correlate with the experts' risk advice (based on evidence) at all. Some patients elected for warfarin when expert evidence suggested that it was unnecessary, and others declined warfarin when expert advice recommended it. Thus individuals all had different ideas about the level of acceptable risk.

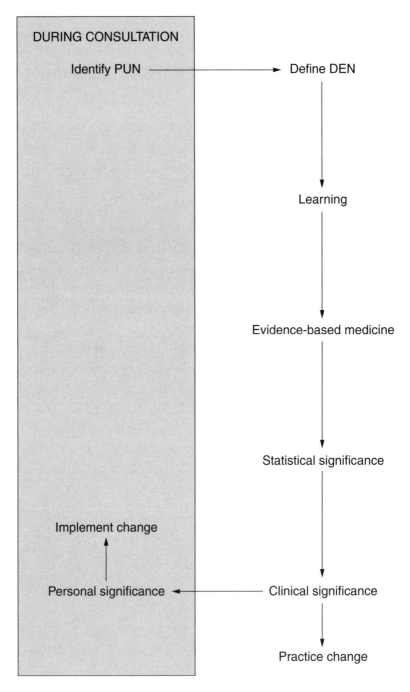

Figure 5.1: Applying evidence-based medicine to personal care.

Bringing best practice to individuals involves not only sharing knowledge but also exploring an individual's understanding of risk. We find patients who want everything that modern medicine can offer to reduce their risk, patients who don't wants pills and 'feel lucky', patients who want you to decide for them, and patients whose intellectual limitations are such that in reality they do need your guidance. In Chapter 1 we considered the approach of a number of different doctors to treating heart failure with ACE inhibitors. We can now see that best practice in the hands of a 'good doctor' does not produce the best statistics.

In summary, when cumulative research produces significant evidence that a particular treatment will benefit a specific population, becoming aware of that information is only the beginning of our journey (*see* Figure 5.1). If we are to make learning useful, we have to do a lot more than merely accumulate knowledge. Turning scientific evidence into clinical and personal significance requires all of the skills that make a good doctor. Without the skills that are necessary to implement change in our practices and in the consulting-room, our knowledge is meaningless.

Reference

1 Protheroe J, Fahey T, Montgomery A *et al.* (2000) The impact of patients' preferences on the treatment of atrial fibrillation: observational study of patient based decision analysis. *BMJ.* **320**: 1380–4.

Chapter 6

Sharing PUNs and DENs

Once you have collected a number of PUNs and described them in your logbook, it is time to set out a learning plan and to have some fun sharing your PUNs with others. New principals seem to have no difficulty in collecting PUNs, as it is still natural for them to be reflective about their work. Long-established principals collect more cautiously, as some of them have forgotten how to reflect on what they were doing. I know many doctors who have rekindled an interest in their work by collecting PUNs, reflection being the key ingredient of lifelong learning.

Arrange your meeting with colleagues and find two hours of protected time. The core group in our practice consists of the doctors, practice nurses and counsellor. You should also invite the practice manager to attend. If you decide to make any changes in practice organisation, the manager will then also 'own' any changes and be able to implement them. Furthermore, practice managers need as much insight as possible into clinical medicine and into what you really think and do.

Someone will need to lead the meeting, but they won't need any special skills. Ask the manager to write some notes so that he or she can produce a summary of the meeting and any group decisions that are made. You can later put this in your personal development plan together with your DENs. Start by

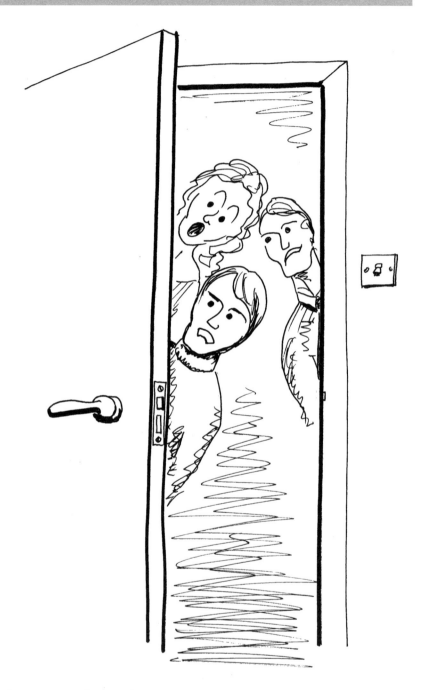

Awareness of what doctors really do behind the consulting room door . . .

taking it in turns to share any clinical knowledge PUNs that you have found, and write them on a flip-chart. Allow the discussion to flow and ensure that everyone has contributed something. You can then move on and share non-clinical knowledge, skills and attitudes. With regard to sharing attitudes, make sure that this is always voluntary and that no one is under pressure to expose themselves. You will discover that colleagues have knowledge you never knew they had, as well as difficulties in areas that will surprise you. At the end of the meeting you should try to outline a plan of learning or change, which can be divided into the following sections.

- *Define some DENs (personal learning needs that you are going to meet on your own).* I have had great fun with my PUN due to lack of knowledge of RAST tests and nut allergy. It seems that my partners (even the 'expert' who used to run an allergy clinic) knew no more than me. A chat with a local consultant was interesting – I felt that peanut allergy was a paediatrician's heartsink. He sent me an excellent paper which basically showed that RAST testing was very unreliable and essentially of no value. I am now collecting literature from numerous allergy support groups.

- *Discover shared DENs, NENs (nurses' educational needs) or even PCTENs (primary care team educational needs).* Whenever we have a PUNs meeting, someone always has a PUN for which we all share the need to learn more. Recently we identified a common desire to understand spirometry and chronic obstructive pulmonary disease. We discovered that our practice nurse with an interest in this area felt isolated and frustrated by the doctors' inconsistent approach. We therefore scheduled a meeting to address the topic. Now all of the doctors and nurses understand it, and we have a respiratory clinic, an agreed protocol and a system for auditing the clinic activity (so often protocols and audits are regarded as threats coming from outside the practice, but because this was PUN based, we 'owned' these and actually wanted them).

- *Agree on delegation.* I once shared a PUN about a demented, chair-bound elderly woman in a nursing home where the staff were convinced that she was suffering with pain from her severely deformed arthritic knees – not an easy assessment, as meaningful communication was long gone. One of my partners offered to visit and managed to find a way of getting a needle into each knee, injecting steroids and providing pain relief. He has since perfected his skill and will inject anything (carpal tunnel is now routine, and he even does finger joints). It was the sharing of PUNs that encouraged us to work as a team, and that gave my partner the confidence to develop his specific skill. Sharing PUNs encourages delegation, skill sharing and teamwork.

- *Practice organisation.* Our poor manager has been very busy since we took up PUN sharing, whether it be auditing or restructuring appointment systems or ensuring that consulting-rooms are properly equipped. The greatest change in management has been an increased awareness of what doctors really do behind the consulting-room door, and balancing the needs of an efficient business with those of good clinical care.

Collecting PUNs is not hard work, and sharing them is fun. If you arrange a two-hour meeting, you will find that there is still plenty of material left to share, and you may want to book a subsequent date to continue with it. You will have started your personal development plan (PDP) and probably got material for your practice professional development plan (PPDP). The main obstacle to getting started is finding the time for the meeting, but once you realise the importance and value of sharing PUNs, I am confident that you will find the time.

Chapter 7

From PUNs and DENs to PDPs

If you have completed a PUNs and DENs exercise, do you have a personal development plan? The answer is most certainly yes. Don't be irritated by PDPs. They do not represent yet more pointless bureaucracy that is being thrust upon you. They are 'personal' (they belong to you), 'developmental' (there are no outcome demands, but an ongoing process to take at your own pace) and a 'plan' (yes, a suggestion that perhaps we would benefit from becoming a little better organised in our learning).

An awareness of the need to have a personal development plan is now well established. At a recent meeting that I attended, two main problems (apart from time and resources) were identified. One was the discomfort of recognising this vacuum and not knowing how to start to fill it. The other was a request for someone to sort it out for them (to tell them what to do, give them some boxes to tick or hurdles to jump, or best described as 'give me the tree on which to hang things'). Well, personal development plans are just that – personal. Each individual's tree will be different. PUNs and DENs is an excellent way to get started. It forms the central trunk from which you can grow.

Starting your PDP

First go out and buy a lever-arch file. Stick a large label on the front saying 'PDP', with your name on it, and you're on the way! Next carry out the PUNs and DENs exercise as described earlier. If you do this and share it with colleagues, you will have defined some relevant personal learning needs. Include in the logbook your plan for meeting these needs. Depending on how much material you collect and how much time you have for learning you can repeat the exercise, say, every six months. You now have a pretty reasonable PDP – you can show anyone that you are reflective, you have considered your learning needs and you have done something about them.

Box 7.1: Short cut to a personal development plan

1 Buy a lever-arch file.
2 Stick a large label on it saying 'PDP'.
3 Write your name on it.
4 Complete PUNs and DENs and add them to the file.

Padding out your PDP

Just remembering to write down those educational activities that are already taking place will add plenty of substance. Jotting down a note about a discussion with a colleague over a cup of coffee adds 'evidence' of learning. File your PGEA certificates at the back. If you read an article in the *British Medical Journal*, the *Journal of the Royal College of General*

Practitioners or the 'medical comics', jot it down. If you have any clinical meetings, make sure that you obtain a copy of the minutes. Nowadays, much clinical governance activity will be going on in your practice, and most of it will no doubt be organised by your practice manager. Make sure that you obtain copies of this for your PDP. Remember to add your PACT data and copies of any audits that are going on in the practice.

Box 7.2: Padding out your PDP

1 What you are already doing.
2 PGEA certificates.
3 Notes on reading.
4 Minutes of clinical meetings.
5 'Bumf' from meetings.
6 Clinical governance activity.
7 PACT data and copies of audits.

Your PDP: getting posh

Next I would suggest that you find out about yourself and what type of learning suits you. Get hold of Honey and Mumford's Learning Styles questionnaire (any GP tutor or course organiser will be able to get you a copy easily). Don't do it on your own, but share it with colleagues – it is useful to know how your partners learn best as well. As a 'reflectionist/activist', the way in which I expressed ideas was often negatively received by a partner. I would have a great idea and I would be thinking that everyone was on board when one of my partners would suddenly let me down and question everything. When I discovered that he was a pure 'theorist', I

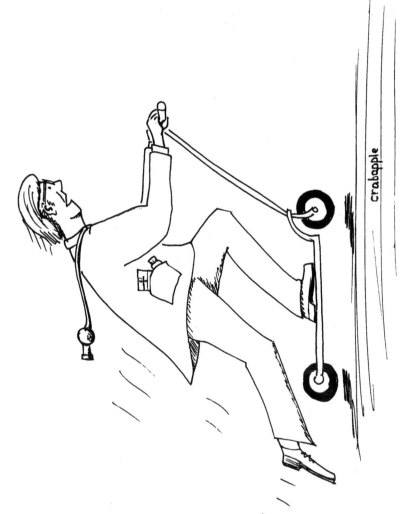

crabapple

The activist.

realised the need to express my ideas differently and offer them in a clear stepwise logical progression. Our ability to communicate effectively has improved enormously as a result. Looking at how you contribute to a team is often useful, and revisiting 'Belbin' can be productive. Make sure that you include your nurses and managers. You may discover that natural chairmanship skills lie with your practice nurse, and that your senior partner has none at all!

Box 7.3: PDP: getting posh

1 Do learning styles.
2 Do 'Belbin'.
3 Psychometric testing.
4 Peer review.
5 Patient questionnaires.
6 Yearly 'away-days'.

You are now beginning to collect material in your PDP file, and you may want to divide it into sections. You may find that it works for you to have four main sections: my needs assessment; me as a person; me as a doctor; me as part of a team.

Significant event audit

This has become popular with appraisers, clinical governance leads and primary care trusts. Of course every PUN that is discovered is a significant event audit. Some organisations have specific formats for recording them. Write out some of your PUNs in this way and you can impress!

Needs assessment

PUNs and DENs work well, but you may want to explore other ways of discovering your learning needs. Do you remember those enormous checklists you had as a registrar, where you tick off how much you know? You may identify some areas that you want to brush up on, but be careful not to tick just the bits you like! You may want to do a type of self-audit. Write down some notes about your career to date, and think about where you want it to go next. Do any learning needs become apparent? You may want to do a Strengths, Weaknesses, Opportunities, Threats (SWOT) analysis either alone or with colleagues. Are you brave enough for a 'peer review'? The different ways of doing this range from a chat with a trusted colleague or your practice manager to full-blown scoring systems from the collection of anonymous data. A system is described in Appendix 2. You might want to draw up a computer-based phased evaluation plan with the Royal College of General Practitioners. You might ask someone to shadow you for a day and tell you want they think. There are many different ways of discovering your learning and development needs, and your local GP tutor should be able to provide you with resources. My poor partners have had to endure peer assessment programmes, team-working assessment and psychometric testing, but don't rush at it and become overwhelmed. Dip your toe in the water and start where you feel most comfortable.

In our practice we all keep our personal development plans differently (one partner keeps it all on his laptop). We all have different subsections. If you have a speciality (e.g. clinical assistant), you will have a section on that. Some of us have sections in which to record activity at self-directed learning groups outside the practice. One partner has a special section for recording their progress in computer skills.

Some actually keep relevant resources such as journal articles in their personal development plan, while others just reference it. When we have in-house educational meetings, we use the first 20 minutes to update and review our PDPs. My own target is to have a PDP with 14 sections, each relating to a different defined area of competence (of which clinical knowledge is only one), but I am in no hurry – my PDP grows with me.

Box 7.4: PDP: showing off

1 Divide your PDP into 14 sections of competence.
2 Assess your needs in each section.
3 Outline ongoing programme to meet your educational needs.
4 Document your success in meeting those needs.
5 Get patient participation groups to review your PDP.

Some doctors feel overwhelmed when they think about creating a PDP. You are not meant to sit down with a mentor, discover and record all of your weaknesses and set out a plan on how to become 'superdoc' by the end of the year. All you need is a little organisation to record what you are probably doing anyway. Remember that learning is life-long. There is no end-point to be reached – it is the direction of travel that is important. So go and buy that lever-arch file, collect some PUNs and watch your own personal learning tree start to grow.

Appendix 1

Discovering learning needs by asking patients

CFEP
Client-Focused Evaluation Programme
Cost: £50
Contact: Julie McGovern
           39 Argyll Road
           Exeter EX4 4RX
           Tel: 01392 252740
           Email: cfep@dialstart.net
           Website: http://latis.ex.ac.uk/cfep

On receipt of the fee you will be sent 50 questionnaires for each doctor, for your patients to complete after their consultation. They are then sent back and you will receive an analysis of what they had to say. In our practice, our practice manager managed to run the whole programme without the doctors knowing about it, so we were unable to be especially pleasant and were caught 'in the raw'. However, it would probably be difficult to keep up a front for 50 consecutive consultations!

Discovering learning needs by asking colleagues

Competency peer review

Introduction

Asking your colleagues whether they think that you are a good doctor can be hazardous. Great care must be taken to carry out the exercise according to the rules. However, discovering what your peers regard as your strengths and weaknesses can bring enormous benefits. Not only will identified weaknesses help you to define your learning needs for your PDP, but identified strengths will give you the confidence to take the lead in various practice activities.

Who assesses you?

You may only want fellow doctors to assess you. In our practice we were each assessed by four partners, two practice managers, one practice nurse and our practice counsellor. The assessments by the non-doctors carried the same weight as those by the doctors. You could ask any members of the primary care team to participate, or even patients, but participants must be able to read and understand the nature of the 14 competencies and know you well enough to form an opinion.

The process

1 All participants were given a copy of the competencies and then had to complete the chart to score all of their partners. They did not score themselves. Each competency was scored on a scale of 1–7.

2 These scores were handed in to an independent adjudicator who added up each doctor's score for each competency and produced an average score. The charts revealing what scores we each gave were destroyed. The adjudicator was now left with a sheet for each doctor, recording their average score for each competency. They then numbered them from 1 for the highest score to 14 for the lowest. Participants never saw their actual scores (so you couldn't tot up who won or who was the best doctor), but only the competencies in the order in which they were most valued by their colleagues. In this way everyone had areas that were most valued.

3 You need to set up an appropriate meeting to hand out the results of the assessment. We used the

first session of our 'away-day'. It is important that this meeting is properly chaired. Each participant received a sheet with their competencies scored in order of value, and was given time to reflect on their results. A column marked 'own value' was used for participants to mark an arrow against each value if they felt that their score was either disappointingly low or too high up the list. Still working independently, they each answered the two questions.

4 It was now time to share some of the results. Competency score sheets remained confidential. We shared our highest and lowest scoring competencies, and from this the group worked together well. Everyone felt valued because everyone had a top competency. It made it very easy for us to share out different leadership roles in the practice. We also shared our weakest competencies without feeling threatened, and all of us planned to address our weakest areas.

5 The exercise produced material for our individual personal development plans and helped to define our roles in the practice. I was most valued for my communication skills. This gave me the confidence to take the lead on education in the practice. I felt that I had been given permission to develop this for the practice. My worst score was for 'job's relationship to society and family'. I felt that they were telling me to stop being a workaholic and to 'get a life'. As a result, I went out and bought a boat!

Competencies

Empathy and sensitivity

Atmosphere in which the patient feels that they are being taken seriously and treated with sensitivity. The doctor is in control, empathetic but not dominating, and the patient feels that they can trust the doctor.

Team involvement

Dealing with colleagues in the partnership. Colleagues are seen as a source of social support. Trust among partners, with no one being too individualistic. Seeing themselves as part of a larger organisation, being able to compromise and show sensitivity to colleagues.

Personal organisation and administrative skills

This includes time management, use of computers, financial skills and knowing when to delegate and how to prioritise.

Stress coping mechanisms

Being aware of own limitations and not keeping things bottled up. Sharing the load with others. Having the ability to switch off and having an interest outside medicine.

Communication skills

Active listening skills, learning to appreciate and notice body language. Learning how to question and to delve deeper. Having humility and empathy. Learning to say sorry and to control one's anger.

Legal, ethical and political awareness

Being aware of the legal/ethical implications of actions but treating the patient in terms of the appropriate clinical route, rather than bowing to market pressures. Trying to cover one's back at all times and having sufficient awareness to protect oneself at all times – safety-netting. Developing lobbying skills at both local and national level and being aware of hidden agendas in Government policy making.

Personal attributes

This is essentially a list of 'trait'-type descriptions for a 'good GP'. They include integrity, flexibility (in action and thoughts), unselfishness, decisiveness, innovative approach, motivation, empathy, warmth, passion and idealism.

Professional integrity

This involves having the courage of one's convictions and acting on those convictions and taking responsibility. The ability to be enthusiastic about the job and to appreciate it when it all works out well.

Conceptual thinking

This involves thinking beyond the obvious. The use of lateral thinking. Being able to judge what is important information from a large mass of information.

Job's relationship to society and family

Respect for those whom society does not like. Putting patients' and family needs before your own.

Personal development

Dealing with how the GP's role has changed and is constantly changing (compare managerial and financial skills). The need to update clinical skills and learn computing skills.

Clinical knowledge

Trust in one's own and others' clinical judgement. Does not over-visit and allow the patient to develop a dependency. Keeps up with current practice and tries to anticipate rather than react.

Managing others

This involves being a skilled negotiator, and a good facilitator (not a dictator). Building bridges between people and motivating them. Being a team player who can work in large groups and participate in decision making.

Learning and development

Willing and able to learn from experience.

Competency	Doctors				TOTAL
	A	B	C	D	
1					
2					
3					
4					
5					
6					
7					
8					
9					
10					
11					
12					
13					
14					
Total					

Do not complete your own score.
1 = very poor, 2 = weak, 3 = rather weak, 4 = acceptable or unable to judge, 5 = good,
6 = very good, 7 = excellent.

A 'good doctor' is competent in the following areas.

Area	Valued by peers	Own value
Empathy and sensitivity		
Team involvement		
Personal organisation and administrative skills		
Stress coping mechanisms		
Communication skills		
Legal, ethical and political awareness		
Personal attributes		
Professional integrity		
Conceptual thinking		
Job's relationship to society and family		
Personal development		
Clinical knowledge		
Managing others		
Learning and development		

1   Areas that I would like to strengthen, or that I recognise the need to strengthen include the following:

2   Areas that interest me, or in which I am already skilled, that I would like to develop and take the lead on include the following:

PUNs summary and logbook

PUN = patient's unmet need   DISCOVERY   DEN = doctor's educational need

1 After each consultation ask yourself *'Was I equipped to meet the patient's needs or could I have done better?'*

2 If you find a PUN, record it on the Discovery page.

3 Also record the following:

- date of consultation
- patient's details
- from the PUN, define the area that is in need of development, improvement or change
- record the class: KC = knowledge clinical
                     KN = knowledge non-clinical
                     S = skill
                     A = attitude

Remember that the Discovery page is confidential to you

THE PROCESS

4 The discoveries highlighted on the Discovery page must now be translated into an educational plan. You may either delegate, define your personal DEN or outline a plan for practice change, development or improvement. (Do not succumb to 'required changes are out of my control' (e.g. unsatisfactory waiting-list for secondary care). Think how you or your practice could influence change.)

5 Finally, complete the action taken. For a complete portfolio do not just include personal learning, but add practice changes as well. Remember that learning with PUNs is personal, non-threatening, starts in the consulting-room and responds to the needs of your patients.

Additional blank templates can be downloaded from www.radcliffe-oxford.com/punsanddens.

CONFIDENTIAL

ASSESSMENT OF EDUCATIONAL NEEDS

PERSONAL PORTFOLIO

LEARNING WITH PUNs AND DENs

Name: ....

DISCOVERY PAGE

CONFIDENTIAL

Date	Patient			The PUN	Define area for improvement, development or change	Class KC/KN/S/A
	No.	Age	Sex			

PROCESS PAGE

The education plan *Define personal DEN/Practice development plan, etc.*	Action taken	Date action completed

DISCOVERY PAGE

Date	Patient			The PUN	Define area for improvement, development or change	Class KC/KN/S/A
	No.	Age	Sex			

PROCESS PAGE

The education plan *Define personal DEN/Practice development plan, etc.*	Action taken	Date action completed

Index